DIABETES MEAL PLAN AND COOKBOOK

For Newly Diagnosed

A 7-Days meal plan To Manage Type 2 Diabetes

BENSON BRAIN

Table of contents

Chapter Seven

Get started with the 7-day Diabetes meal plan

Introduction

Being diagnosed with diabetes is a life-changing event, but it doesn't mean you can't live a happy and healthy life. Treating diabetes requires constant care and attention. Although it will probably be very overwhelming at first, over time you will develop a better idea of how to manage the condition and be in harmony with your body.

It's hard to know where to start, what to believe, and how to make changes to your routine. As with most health changes, we want to make a habit. The trick is to start small.

Maybe start by replacing one sugary drink with water each day, increasing the number of drinks you replace until you have replaced most or all. Incorporated more home-cooked meals, starting with one meal at a time if you eat out often. Also consider adding more fruits, non-starchy vegetables, lean proteins, and whole grains to your plate (which is exactly what you'll see in this meal plan).

If you've recently been diagnosed with type 2 diabetes but are now ready to change your diet, the prospect of giving up the foods you love may seem daunting. But you may be relieved to discover that eating well with type 2 diabetes is not as difficult as you think and that you can still enjoy food despite treating the disease. A healthy diet is the cornerstone of a successful diabetes management plan. Other pillars include managing stress, exercising regularly, and taking prescribed medications.

Chapter One

What is diabetes?

Diabetes is a disease that occurs when the level of sugar (glucose) in the blood is too high. It occurs when the pancreas does not produce enough insulin or when the body does not respond properly to the effects of insulin.

The hormone insulin transports sugar from the blood to cells, where it is stored or used for energy. If this doesn't work, you may have diabetes.

Untreated high blood sugar due to diabetes can damage nerves, eyes, kidneys, and other organs. But by educating yourself about diabetes and taking steps to prevent or treat it, you can protect your health.

Types of diabetes

There are different types of diabetes:

•Type 1 Diabetes
Type 1 diabetes is when the immune system attacks and destroys the cells of the pancreas, where insulin is produced. It is unclear what caused this attack.it is an autoimmune disease

•Type 2: Type 2 diabetes occurs when your body develops insulin resistance and sugar builds up in the blood. It is the most common type about 90 to 95% of people with diabetes have type 2.

•Type 1.5: Type 1.5 diabetes is also known as latent autoimmune diabetes in adults (LADA). It occurs in adulthood and, like type 2 diabetes, has a gradual onset. LADA is an autoimmune disease that cannot be treated through diet or lifestyle.

•Gestational diabetes: Gestational diabetes is high blood sugar levels during pregnancy. This type of diabetes is caused by insulin- blocking hormones produced by the placenta.

A condition called diabetes insipidus not related to diabetes mellitus, although it has a similar name. It is another condition in which the kidneys remove too much fluid from the body.

Each type of diabetes has unique symptoms, causes and treatment options.

•Prediabetes

Prediabetes occurs when the blood sugar level is higher than expected, but not high enough to diagnose type 2 diabetes. It occurs when the body's cells do not respond to insulin as they should.

Experts estimate that more than one in three Americans has prediabetes, but more than 80% of people with prediabetes don't even know it.

•Diabetes symptoms

Diabetes symptoms are caused by increased blood sugar.

General symptoms

The symptoms of type 1, type 2 and type 1.5 (LADA) are the same but occur over a shorter period than types 2 and 1.5. Type 2 tends to have a slower onset. Tingling nerves and slow-healing wounds are more common in type 2.

Type 1 in particular can cause diabetic ketoacidosis if left untreated. This occurs when there are dangerous levels of ketones in the body. It is less common with other types of diabetes, but still possible.

•Common symptoms of diabetes include:

•Increased hunger

• Increased thirst

•Weight Loss

•Frequent urination

•Blurry vision

•Feel Exhausted

•Wounds that do not heal

Symptoms in men
The common symptoms in men with diabetes may include:

•A reduced sexual desire

•Erectile dysfunction

•little muscle strength

Symptoms in women.
Women with diabetes may experience the following symptoms:

•Vaginal dryness

•Urinary tract infection

•Fungal infections

•Itchy dry skin

Gestational Diabetes
Most people who develop gestational diabetes do not have symptoms. Health professionals usually detect the condition during a routine blood glucose test or oral glucose tolerance test, which is usually performed between 24 and 28 weeks of pregnancy.

In rare cases, a person with gestational diabetes may also experience increased thirst or urination.

Chapter Two

Causes of diabetes

Each type of diabetes has different associated causes.

Diabetes type 1
What's the exact cause of type 1 diabetes is not know.The immune system accidentally attacks and destroys the insulin-producing beta cells in the pancreas.

Genetics also plays a role in some people. There is also a possibility for a virus to trigger an attack on the immune system.

•Type 2 diabetes

Type 2 diabetes occurs due to a combination of genetic and lifestyle factors. Being overweight also increases the risk.

Carrying extra weight, especially in the abdominal area, makes cells more resistant to the effects of insulin on blood sugar.

This condition tends to run in families. Family members share genes that increase the risk of developing type 2 diabetes and being overweight.

Diabetes type 1.5

Type 1.5 is an autoimmune disease that occurs when the pancreas is attacked by its own antibodies. As in type 1. It may be genetic, but more research is required.

Gestational diabetes
Gestational diabetes occurs because of hormonal changes during pregnancy.
The placenta produces hormones that make the person's pregnant cells less sensitive to the effects of insulin.
This can cause high blood sugar levels during pregnancy.

People who are overweight or gain too much weight during pregnancy have a higher risk of developing gestational diabetes.

•Diabetes risk Factors
Certain factors increase your risk of diabetes.

Diabetes type 1
You are more likely to develop type 1 diabetes if you are a child or teenager, if a parent or sibling has the disease, or if you carry certain genes linked to the disease.

Type 2 diabetes

You might be at the risk of type 2 diabetes if you:

•Overweight

•Are at least 45 years old

•Have a parent or sibling who suffers from this disease

•They are not physically active

•Had gestational diabetes

•You have prediabetes

• High blood pressure and high cholesterol.

Type 2 diabetes also affects certain racial and ethnic populations disproportionately.

According to a research in 2016, adults of African American or Asian American, Latinos descent are more likely to be diagnosed with type 2 diabetes than white adults. They are also more likely to experience poorer quality of care and greater barriers to self-management.

Diabetes type 1.5

Type 1.5 diabetes occurs in adults over 30 years of age and is often confused with type 2 diabetes. However, people with this condition are not necessarily overweight and oral medications and lifestyle changes have no effect.

Gestational diabetes

Your risk of gestational diabetes increases if you:

•Are overweight

• Are over 25 years old

•Had gestational diabetes during a previous pregnancy

•Have given birth to a baby who weighs more than 9 pounds.

•Type 2 diabetes runs in the family

•Has polycystic ovary syndrome (PCOS).

Chapter Three

Complications and treatment of diabetes.

High blood sugar levels damage organs and tissues throughout the body. The higher your blood sugar level and the longer you live with it, the higher your risk of complications.

Complications associated with diabetes include:

•Heart diseases, heart attacks and strokes.

•Neuropathy

•Nephropathy

•Retinopathy and vision loss.

•Hearing loss

•Damage to the feet, such as Infections and wounds that do not heal

•Skin diseases such as fungal and bacterial infections

•Depression

•Dementia

Gestational Diabetes
Untreated gestational diabetes can cause problems that affect both mother and child. Complications affecting the baby may include:

•Premature birth

•Birth weight higher than normal

•Risk of type 2 diabetes increase in the future

•Low blood sugar

•Jaundice

•Birth of a stillborn child

A pregnant person may develop complications such as high blood pressure or type 2 diabetes due to gestational diabetes. They may also need a cesarean section, commonly called a C-section.

It also increases the risk of gestational diabetes in future pregnancies.

Diabetes treatment

Doctors treat diabetes with various medications. Some are taken orally, others are available as injections.

The four key aspects of diabetes treatment include:

Blood sugar monitoring: Monitoring your blood sugar (glucose) level is key to determining how well your current treatment plan is working. It gives you daily (and sometimes even hourly) information on how to manage your diabetes. You can monitor your levels by checking regularly with a finger-stick glucose meter and/or a continuous glucose monitor (CGM). You and your doctor will determine the best blood sugar range for you.

Oral diabetes medications: Oral diabetes medications (taken by mouth) help control blood sugar levels in people who have diabetes but still produce some insulin, mainly people with type 2 diabetes and prediabetes. People with gestational diabetes may also need oral medications. There are different types. Metformin is the most common.

Insulin: People with type 1 diabetes need to inject synthetic insulin to live and control diabetes. Some people with type 2 diabetes also need insulin. There are different types of synthetic insulin. Each starts working at different speeds and stays in your body for different periods. The four major ways to administer insulin include syringe injectable insulin (insulin syringe), insulin pens, insulin pumps, and rapid-acting inhaled insulin.

Diet: Meal planning and choosing a healthy diet are important aspects of diabetes management because foods have a major impact on blood sugar. If you take insulin, counting carbohydrates in the foods and drinks you eat is an important part of treatment. The amount of carbohydrates you eat determines how much insulin you need at meals. Healthy eating habits can also help you control your weight and reduce your risk of heart disease.

Exercise: Physical activity increases insulin sensitivity (and helps reduce insulin resistance), so regular exercise is an important part of treatment for all people with diabetes.

Due to the increased risk of heart disease, it is also important to maintain a healthy diet:
Weight.

Blood pressure.

Cholesterol.

•Diabetes types 1 and 1.5
Insulin is the main treatment for type 1 and type 1.5 diabetes. Replaces the hormone that your body cannot produce.

People with type 1 and type 1.5 diabetes often use different types of insulin. They differ in the speed with which they act and the duration of their effect:

•Rapid-acting insulin: it begins to act in 15 minutes and its effects last 2 to 4 hours.

•Short-acting insulin: begins to act in 30 minutes and lasts 3 to 6 hours.

•Intermediate-acting insulin: begins to act in 2 to 4 hours and lasts 12 to 18 hours.

•Long-acting insulin: begins to act 2 hours after injection and lasts up to 24 hours.

•Ultra-long-acting insulin: begins to act 6 hours after injection and lasts 36 hours or more.

•Premixed insulin: Starts working in 15 to 30 minutes (depending on whether the mixture includes rapid-acting or short-acting insulin) and lasts 10 to 16 hours.

•Type 2 Diabetes

Diet and exercise can help some people control type 2 diabetes. If lifestyle changes are not enough to lower blood sugar, you will need to take medication.

•Gestational Diabetes
If you are diagnosed with gestational diabetes, you will need to check your blood sugar levels several times a day during pregnancy. If the level is high, changes in diet and exercise may be enough to reduce it.

Research shows that about 15 to 30% of women who have gestational diabetes need insulin to lower blood sugar. Insulin is safe for the developing baby.

Diabetes and nutrition

Healthy eating is a central part of diabetes treatment. In some cases, a change in diet may be enough to control the disease.

Diabetes types 1 and 1.5

Your blood sugar levels rise or fall depending on the type of food you eat. Starchy or sugary foods cause blood sugar levels to rise quickly. Proteins and fats cause a more gradual increase.

Your healthcare team may recommend that you limit the amount of carbohydrates you eat each day. It is also necessary to balance carbohydrate intake with insulin doses. Counting carbs helps balance carbohydrate intake with insulin doses.

Type 2 diabetes

Eating the right foods can control blood sugar levels and help you lose excess weight.

Counting carbohydrates is an important part of the type 2 diabetes diet. A nutritionist can help you determine how many grams of carbohydrates you should consume at each meal.

To keep your blood sugar levels stable, try to eat small meals throughout the day. Emphasize healthy foods such as:

•Fruit

•Vegetables

•Grain

•Lean proteins such as fish and poultry.

Certain other foods can interfere with efforts to control blood sugar levels.

Discover the foods you should avoid if you have diabetes.

Gestational diabetes

During these 9 months of pregnancy a balanced diet is very important for you and your baby. Choosing the right foods can also help you avoid taking diabetes medications.

Limit sugary or salty foods and watch your portion size. Although you need sugar for your growing baby, you should avoid eating too much. The right ratio of protein, fat, and carbohydrates can help you control your blood sugar levels.

Chapter Four

Exercises and diabetes diagnosis.

In addition to diet and treatment, exercise plays an essential role in diabetes control. It's applicable to almost all types of diabetes.

When you stay active, your cells respond more effectively to insulin and lower your blood sugar levels. Regular exercise can also help you:

•Achieve and maintain a healthy weight

•Reduce your risk of diabetes-related health complications

•Increase mood

•Sleep better

•Improve memory

If you have type 1 or type 2 diabetes, you should aim to get at least 150 minutes of moderate-intensity exercise each week. There are currently no specific exercise guidelines for people with gestational diabetes. However, if you are pregnant, start slowly and gradually increase your activity level over time to avoid overexertion.

Diabetes-friendly exercises include:

• Walking

• Swimming

• Dancing

• Cycling

Talk to your doctor about safe ways to incorporate activities into your diabetes management plan. You may need to follow special precautions, such as Monitor your blood sugar before and after exercise and make sure you stay hydrated.

Consider working with a personal trainer or exercise physiologist who has experience working with diabetics. They can help you develop an individual training plan tailored to your needs.

Diagnosis of diabetes

Anyone who has symptoms of diabetes or is at risk for the condition should get tested. Women are routinely tested for gestational diabetes in the second or third trimester of pregnancy.

To diagnose prediabetes and diabetes, doctors use these blood tests:

•The fasting plasma glucose (FPG) test measures your blood sugar level after you have fasted for 8 hours.

•The A1C test provides a snapshot of your blood sugar levels over the past 3 months.

•a 75 gram oral glucose tolerance test can also be used. Blood sugar is checked 2 hours after consuming a sugary drink with 75 grams of carbohydrates.

How to diagnose gestational diabetes

To diagnose gestational diabetes, your doctor will test your blood sugar levels between 24 and 28 weeks of pregnancy. There are two types of tests:

•Glucose challenge test: A glucose challenge test checks your blood sugar level one hour after drinking a liquid that contains sugar. If your results are standard, no further testing will be done. If blood sugar levels are high, you will need to undergo a glucose tolerance test.

•Glucose tolerance test: A glucose tolerance test checks the blood sugar level after an overnight fast. They will then give you a sugary drink and measure your blood sugar again after one hour and again after two hours. Gestational diabetes is diagnosed when any of these three values indicate high blood sugar levels.

As soon as you are diagnosed with diabetes, the sooner you can begin the treatment. Find out if you should be tested and learn more about any tests your doctor has performed.

Chapter five

Diabetes prevention

Type 1 and type 1.5 diabetes cannot be prevented because they are caused by a disorder of the immune system. Some causes of type 2 diabetes, such as genes or age, are also out of your control.

However, many other diabetes risk factors can be controlled. Most diabetes prevention strategies involve simple adjustments to your diet and fitness program.

If you have been diagnosed with prediabetes, here are some things you can do to delay or prevent type 2 diabetes:

•Do aerobic exercise such as walking or cycling for at least 150 minutes per week.

• Eliminate saturated and trans fats and refined carbohydrates from your diet.

•Eat vegetables,whole grains and more fruits

•Eat smaller portions.

Aim to lose 5 to 7% of your body weight if you are overweight.

These are not the only ways to prevent diabetes. Discover other strategies that can help you avoid this chronic health condition.

Diabetes in pregnancy

People who have never had diabetes can suddenly develop gestational diabetes during pregnancy. Hormones the placenta produces can make your body more resistant to the effects of insulin.

Pregestational diabetes

People can have diabetes before they become pregnant and pass it on during pregnancy. This is called pregestational diabetes.

Risks for your newborn

Diabetes during pregnancy can cause complications such as jaundice or breathing problems in the newborn.

If you are diagnosed with pregestational or gestational diabetes, you will need special monitoring to prevent complications.

Does gestational diabetes go away on its own?

Gestational diabetes should go away after delivery, but it significantly increases the risk of developing diabetes later in life. About half of people with gestational diabetes develop type 2 diabetes.

Diabetes in children

Children can also get this type 1 and type 2 diabetes. Controlling blood sugar is particularly important in young people because diabetes can damage important organs such as the heart and kidneys.

Diabetes type 1

The autoimmune form of diabetes usually begins in childhood. One of the major symptoms is increased urination. Children with type 1 diabetes may begin to wet the bed after using the bathroom.

Extreme thirst, tiredness, and hunger are also signs of the disease. Children with type 1 diabetes must receive immediate treatment. The condition can cause high blood sugar, dehydration, and diabetic ketoacidosis (DKA), which can constitute a medical emergency.

Type 2 diabetes

Type 1 diabetes was previously called juvenile diabetes because type 2 diabetes was very rare in children. As more children become overweight, type 2 diabetes becomes more common in this age group.

Some children with type 2 diabetes do not experience any symptoms. Others may experience:

• Increased thirst

•Frequent urination

•Exhausted

•Blurry vision

Type 2 diabetes is often diagnosed based on medical history, a physical exam, and blood tests.

Untreated type 2 diabetes can cause lifelong complications, such as heart disease, kidney disease, and blindness. Healthy eating and exercise can help your child control their blood sugar levels and prevent these problems.

Type 2 diabetes is more common among young people. Learn to recognize the signs so you can report them to your child's doctor.

Chapter six

Meal planning for diabetics.

Meal plan for everyday of the week.

Carbohydrate counting and the plate method are two common tools that can help you plan your meals.

A nutrition plan is your guide to when, what, and how much you should eat to get the nutrients you need while keeping your blood sugar levels within your target range. A good nutrition plan takes into account your goals, tastes and lifestyle, as well as the medications you take.

So what is a good diet for type 2 diabetes?

•The DASH diet

The DASH (Dietary Approaches to Stop Hypertension) diet is a low-sodium plan that promotes a healthy diet to reduce high blood pressure. The DASH diet contains foods rich in potassium, magnesium, and calcium. Saturated fat, sodium, and sugar are limited because they can raise blood sugar, blood pressure, and LDL cholesterol, which are major risks for heart disease and stroke. DASH limits sodium intake to 2,300 mg per day.

That's about the same amount of sodium as in a can of concentrated chicken noodle soup or a teaspoon of table salt.

For those who need to reduce their sodium intake, there is a DASH diet with an even more restrictive sodium recommendation (1500 mg per day).

•Mediterranean diet

The Mediterranean diet has become popular in the United States. It is a nutritional approach that enhances foods traditionally consumed in Mediterranean countries such as France, Greece, Spain and Italy.

This diet is rich in healthy fats such as extra virgin olive oil and includes fruits and vegetables, whole grains, nuts, seeds, and fatty fish such as salmon. Eggs and cheese are consumed in moderation. processed foods,red meat and refined oils and grains are rarely eaten.

Studies have shown that people with diabetes who follow a Mediterranean diet have less insulin resistance and lower A1C levels (a test that measures blood sugar over the past three months). Furthermore, according to another study, the Mediterranean diet can protect the cognitive functions of the brain. That could mean:

Improved memory

Higher processing speed

Low risk of neurological diseases such as dementia and Alzheimer's

This approach reminds us that the best "diet" for controlling diabetes is not just a diet, but a lifestyle change.

•Foods for type 2 diabetics

Portion control and carbohydrate counting are essential no matter what foods you choose. If you're not familiar with portion sizes, portion control can seem subjective. You may find portion sizes confusing.

•Serving Sizes

You can illustrate serving sizes by hand. Let's look at some examples of foods for each size:

A fingertip portion is approximately one teaspoon. Think of mayonnaise, oils, butter and margarine.

A thumb portion is approximately equal to a tablespoon. Examples of thumb portions are Cheese sticks,nut butter,sour cream and salad dressing.

A handful is approximately one to two ounces. Nuts, pretzels, and crackers fit in the palm of the average-sized hand (2.91 to 3.30 inches, depending on gender) without filling it.

A palm piece weighs 3 to 4 ounces and fits completely in the palm of the hand down to the fingers and thumb. Portion sizes of fish, meat, poultry, pasta, cooked vegetables and potatoes fit into an average palm serving. To get an idea of approximate size, imagine holding a deck of cards in the palm of your hand.

A handful is approximately equal to one cup or eight ounces. It can be a cup of soup, raw vegetables, salad or cereal.

•Plate sizes

Portion sizes in the United States are larger than in Europe. Our plate sizes have grown more than 36% in the last 50 years. We've gone from nine-inch diameter plates to one-foot diameter plates, especially in restaurants where portion sizes are typically two or three times larger than the average portion size.

Now that you have a better understanding of portion and plate sizes, let's look at what types of foods you should eat.

•The glycemic index (GI)
Any food containing carbohydrates can potentially increase your glucose levels. The glycemic index is designed to classify foods

into "low," "medium," and "high" categories on a scale of 1 to 100, based on how quickly they raise blood sugar levels.

Lower values indicate a less chance of your glucose levels rising quickly.

Foods can be classified as follows:

Low glycemic value: GI of 50 or less

Average glycemic value: GI of 50-70

High glycemic index: GI of 70 or more

Foods like packaged and flavored oats typically have a GI of around 80. On the other hand, cut oats lower the GI to 55, making them a better choice for your diet.

•Bread, cereals, and pasta.

Look for whole grains, non-white bread, and whole-grain or vegetable pasta that contain complex rather than simple carbohydrates.

pita bread

Whole-meal bread

Non-instant oatmeal

pasta

Brown rice

Complex carbohydrates take longer to break down than simple carbohydrates, which quickly turn into sugar. Whole grain products are also rich in fiber and make you feel full faster. However, pay attention to portion sizes, as they may also contain more calories.

•Nuts and legumes
Nuts are rich in protein and can be high in calories. Legumes, especially beans, are a

great source of protein, but they tend to be relatively low in calories.

black beans

Pinto beans

Lentils

walnuts

Remember that peanuts and therefore peanut butter are legumes.

•Starchy vegetables

Starch is the type of carbohydrate stored in vegetables. The following starchy vegetables should be consumed in moderation or they will increase your blood sugar levels:

Corn

Peas

potatoes

Squeeze

When it comes to starchy vegetables, choose wisely and practice portion control. Instead of a baked white potato, choose a sweet potato or yam.choose sweet potato fries or baked radish slices instead of French fries

It is not necessary to avoid all "white" foods. You need a variety of foods in your diet.

•Non-starchy vegetables

Low-starch vegetables tend to be dark, leafy, and green, but they can also be light, such as cauliflower and bamboo shoots.

Cruciferous vegetables like broccoli and cabbage contain a lot of water, fiber, and glucosinolate. Glucosinolate is known to inhibit the growth of cancer cells and is effective against inflammatory diseases. They include:

broccoli

Brussels sprouts

zucchini

Mushrooms

Bamboo shoots

Artichoke hearts

Spinach

Cauliflower

Cucumbers

Green beans

Dark-green, leafy vegetables

Root vegetables

To get the most variety in your diet, choose starchy and non-starchy vegetables every day.

•Milk and yogurt

Stick to low-fat dairy products instead of full-fat products. Foods in this category include:

Nut milk

Cow milk

soy milk

Yogurt

Be careful of hidden sugars in flavored dairy products. A single serving of flavored yogurt can contain 40 g of sugar. If you eliminate lactose, the natural sugar, you are left with five to seven teaspoons of hidden sugar.
Fruit

Fruit naturally contains fructose, which causes a smaller rise in blood sugar levels compared to glucose. However, you should include fruits in your diet as they contain fiber and phytochemicals.

Fiber slows down the digestive process and helps relieve blood sugar spikes. Phytochemical stimulates the immune system and slows the growth of cancer cells.

Fruits you can eat include:

Apples

Bananas

Cherries

Dates

Fruit cocktail

Grapes

Kiwi

Melons

Oranges

Peaches

Pears

Prunes

Raisins

Strawberries

Watermelon

Snacks
A good snack satisfies cravings by keeping carbs to a minimum. It's important to incorporate snacks into your meal, planning every day to maintain a variety of your favorite foods.

Some snack ideas include:

Crackers (whole-grain, baked)

French fries (baked)

Popcorn (air-fed or microwaved, no butter)

French fries (whole-grain, baked)

The purpose of snacks should be to normalize blood sugar levels and keep energy levels high.

Sauces and spices
Foods without spices can be very simple, making healthy eating difficult. Sauces and spices should only be a small portion of your diabetic menu.

Some examples are:

Barbecue sauce

fruit jam

Jelly

Honey

Ketchup

Mayonnaise

Mustard

Nut butter

Ranch dressing

Salsa

Sauces

Syrups

"Low sugar" does not mean "calorie-free." Read your labels and choose your extras carefully. Drizzling whole wheat waffles with syrup does not keep blood sugar levels at healthy levels. Try fruit jam for a sweet change or salsa for a savory treat.

•Foods that patients with type 2 diabetes should avoid

People with diabetes should avoid processed foods, such as packaged deli meats, cheese, chips, and ready meals. Other foods to avoid include:

High-fat meats, especially beef, duck, poultry with skin, dark meats.

Fat dairy products such as whole milk,butter and sour cream.

Non-diet soft drinks and fruit juices sweetened with sugar.

Sugar, especially table sugar, honey, molasses, and brown sugar.

Foods are high in trans fats, such as shortening, non-dairy coffee creamers, and anything containing partially hydrogenated oils.

Fried foods, unless you fry them in olive oil or use a deep fryer

If you simply can't live without some of these foods, eat them in moderation and with healthier foods.

•Food labels
When choosing foods for your type 2 diabetes meal plan, it is important to learn to read food labels. This is very important if you have food allergies.

When choosing which foods to include in your diet, read labels for ingredients, carbohydrates, fiber, and fat content.

Ingredients are listed in descending order, with the most used ingredient being the least used.

Look at the total amount of carbohydrates in grams on the label. This breaks down into added sugars, complex carbohydrates, and fiber. Check if the carbohydrates are natural sugars or processed sugars. Natural sugars, such as those found in milk and fruits, are a better choice than the sugars found in cereals. If its label says "sugar free," it doesn't necessarily mean it's carbohydrate free. Sugar-free labels mean that one serving contains less than 0.5g of sugar.

Fat-free foods may still contain carbohydrates. Fat has more than twice as many calories as carbohydrates or sugar. Trans fats and saturated fats can increase cholesterol levels. Choose monounsaturated or polyunsaturated fats, as they are good for your heart.

How can your meal Planning Help You Manage Type 2 Diabetes

Consistency is important in the treatment of diabetes. Meal planning helps you stay consistent in your eating habits while balancing your daily carbohydrate intake. This is especially important if your treatment plan includes insulin injections, as insulin doses may need to be changed based on food intake.

Meal planning also provides a visual representation of how many calories and carbs each food choice contains, whether you make a list manually or record your consumption on an app.

•Benefits of a diabetes meal plan

By recording which foods you eat at each meal, along with portion sizes, calories, and carbs, you can see at a glance which foods go together for breakfast, lunch, dinner, and snacks.

Some doctors may recommend eating up to six smaller meals a day, depending on other medical conditions you may have. If you need to lose weight, your diet plan may include 1,200 to 1,600 calories per day.

The benefits of following your type 2 diabetes eating plan include:

Glucose control

Weight control

Reduced need for diabetes medication

Less risk of heart diseases such as high blood pressure.

Reducing the risk of high cholesterol.

You can include in your diet any food that contains less than 20 calories per serving and less than 5 g of carbohydrates per serving ("free" foods). When it comes to free food, pay attention to portion sizes.

Chapter seven

Get started with the 7-day diabetes meal plan

When it comes to treating type 2 diabetes, developing and maintaining a healthy, balanced diet is the most useful advice.

However, it's also important to pay attention to the type and amount of carbohydrate-containing foods you eat and avoid foods high in unhealthy fats, added sugar, and salt.

Eating a moderate amount of carbohydrate foods with a low glycemic index (GI) can be beneficial, as well as spacing meals evenly throughout the day.

This recommended 7-day meal plan contains recipes that are low to medium GI, low in saturated fat, and high in fiber, making it suitable and beneficial for most people with type 2 diabetes.

Notes on this meal plan

This nutrition plan provides an average of 8,700 kilojoules per day and is based on the average energy needs of adults with diabetes ages 18 to 65. Your energy and nutritional needs vary depending on your age, activity, health, height, and weight.

This meal plan provides the minimum number of servings of each of the major food groups recommended by the U.S. Healthy Eating Guide* for adults (except for women over 51 and men over 70 who may need additional milk, cheese, or yogurt.)

This meal plan requires 9 eggs per week.

Keep in mind that it is also important to drink plenty of water.

•Day One

Breakfast

Porridge: 1/2 cup dry rolled oats with 1 cup skim milk + 1 serving of fruit (e.g. 1 medium banana or 1 orange)

Lunch

Scrambled eggs on toast: 2 eggs scrambled on 2 slices of soy and flaxseed bread, 2 cups of salad greens (e.g. lettuce), ½ avocado, and low-fat cheese.

Dinner

Fried chicken: 100g chicken with 1.5 cups cooked vegetables, 1 cup cooked rice/low GI brown rice, and 2 tsp Oil.

Dessert/dinner

Yogurt with flaxseed: 1 cup of skim yogurt without added sugar with 1 tablespoon of flaxseed.

Appetizers

1 serving of fruit (e.g. 1 medium orange, pear, or apple)

•Day Two

Breakfast

Whole grain cereal: 3/4 cup whole grain cereal with 1 cup low-fat milk + 1 serving of fruit (for example, ¾ cup grapes or 1 medium peach)

Lunch

Grilled fish and vegetables: 125g of grilled fish + 2 cups of steamed vegetables + ½ cup of mashed sweet potato.

+ 1 cup of skimmed yogurt with no added sugar

Dinner

Healthy lentil and feta frittata (1 serving), served with 1 slice of whole wheat bread.

Dessert/dinner

Fruit Salad Dessert: 1 cup fresh fruit salad mixed with ½ cup low-fat Greek yogurt

Appetizers

2 whole grain crackers with avocado spread

•Day Three

Breakfast

Creamy Mushroom Croque Madame (1 serving)

Lunch

Roasted lamb and vegetables: 150 g lean lamb with 1 medium ear of corn, 1.5 cups baked vegetables, and 2 teaspoons oil (for cooking).

+ Bunch of grapes

Dinner

Chicken and Quinoa Salad: 100 g lean chicken + 1 cup cooked quinoa + 2 cups green leafy vegetables + ½ avocado + low-fat cheese + 2 teaspoons oil (for cooking).

Dessert/dinner

Fruit smoothie: 1 cup low-fat milk + 1 serving of fruit (e.g., banana or mixed berries), pureed

Appetizers

a handful of almonds

•Day Four

Breakfast

Granola Yogurt: 1 cup (200 g) low-fat plain yogurt with 1 teaspoon chia/flaxseed flour and ¼ cup dry toasted granola.

+ 1 serving of fruit (e.g. 1 banana or medium pear)

Lunch

Lentil, vegetable, and barley soup: 3/4 cup of lentils with 1 cup of vegetables, vegetable broth, and 1 cup of cooked barley

+ 1 medium whole wheat roll

Dinner

Fried dinner: 120 g lean pork + 1 medium baked sweet potato + 1.5 cups baked vegetables + 2 teaspoons oil (for cooking)

Dessert/dinner

Fresh Fruit and Cheese Platter – Cut up a variety of fresh seasonal fruits and serve with low-fat cheese.

Appetizers

1 cup low-fat yogurt with no added sugar

•Day Five

Breakfast

Mushroom and tomato omelet (1 serving) + 1 glass of skimmed milk/vegetable milk enriched with calcium

Lunch

Tuna and Lettuce Wrap: 100 g canned tuna + 1/2 avocado + 2 cups salad greens (e.g. lettuce, cucumber, carrot, pepper) + 1 slice barley/whole wheat wrap.

+ 1 serving of fruit (for example, 1 medium banana, orange, or 1 cup of mixed berries)

Dinner

Whole Grain Pasta with Tomato: 2/3 cup lean ground beef/pork cooked in tomato sauce with 1 cup cooked whole grain pasta + grated low-fat cheese and 2 teaspoons oil (for cooking)

+ 2 cups of salad (baby spinach, carrots, cucumber, tomatoes)

Dessert/dinner

Yogurt with berries: 1 cup low-fat yogurt with no added sugar with berries and cinnamon

Appetizers

2 whole grain crackers with hummus and cucumber slices

•Day Six

Breakfast

Whole grain muesli: 3/4 cup whole grain muesli + 2 tablespoons of psyllium husks with 1 cup of milk, and 1 tablespoon of flaked almonds.

+ 1 serving of fruit (e.g. ¾ cup of grapes or 2 kiwis)

Lunch

Healthy boiled egg salad (1 serving) + 1 cup of skimmed yogurt with no added sugar.

Dinner

Chicken and Veggie Bowl: Toss together roasted chicken + 1/3 cup chickpeas + crumbled low-fat feta + 2 cups salad greens (e.g., bell pepper, carrot, peas, arugula) + 1 cup rice cooked whole wheat.

Dessert/dinner

Fruit salad: 1 cup fresh fruit salad (for example, strawberries, blueberries, apples, and oranges)

Appetizers

A handful of walnuts.

•Seventh Day

Breakfast

Tomato and Avocado Toast: 1 slice of whole wheat toast with tomato + avocado +

skimmed cheese + 1 glass of skimmed milk/calcium-fortified vegetable milk

Lunch

Chicken and vegetable soup: 100 g lean chicken + 1 cup cooked vegetables (e.g. tomato, celery, carrot) with vegetable broth

Dinner

Salmon, rice and vegetables: 125 g fresh salmon + 1 cup cooked rice/low GI basmati rice + 1.5 cups steamed vegetables + 2 tsp oil (for cooking)

Dessert/dinner

Fruit Pop: Made with frozen fruit (for example, mango or berries) with Greek yogurt.

Appetizers

A bunch of grapes or 1 medium apple

www.ingramcontent.com/pod-product-compliance
Lightning Source LLC
Chambersburg PA
CBHW050846260726
48660CB00006B/2475